CIALIS (TADALAFIL) USAGE GUIDE FOR MEN

**A Balanced Perspective On Using Cialis
For Managing Erectile Dysfunction.**

Kim Bright

DISCLAIMER

Disclaimer

The information provided in this Cialis *Usage Guide* is intended for educational purposes only and should not be construed as medical advice. This guide aims to offer insights into the safe and informed use of Stendra for erectile health. However, it is not a substitute for professional medical consultation, diagnosis, or treatment.

Readers are encouraged to seek the advice of qualified healthcare professionals regarding any medical condition or treatment. The authors and publishers of this guide do not assume any liability for the decisions made based on the information presented herein. All medical treatments should be approached with care and under the guidance of a healthcare provider.

Table Of Contents

Introduction To Cialis

In this guide, we aim to provide a comprehensive understanding of Cialis (tadalafil), a commonly prescribed medication for managing erectile dysfunction (ED) and, in some cases, benign prostatic hyperplasia (BPH). Dealing with ED can be challenging, both physically and emotionally, often impacting self-confidence, relationships, and overall quality of life. This guide seeks to address those challenges by offering clear and reliable information on how Cialis works, the best ways to take it, and what you should know to use it effectively and safely.

Understanding ED involves recognizing the range of factors that contribute to it. These can include cardiovascular issues, diabetes, hormonal imbalances, and lifestyle choices such as smoking and poor diet. Psychological factors, including stress and anxiety, can also play a significant role. The impact of ED goes beyond physical challenges, often affecting mental well-being, intimate relationships, and overall quality of life.

Cialis (tadalafil) is a medication in the phosphodiesterase type 5 (PDE5) inhibitor class and is widely used for managing ED. It works by enhancing blood flow to the penis during sexual stimulation, helping to maintain an erection. Its longer duration of action, often up to 36 hours, allows for flexibility, making it a unique option compared to other ED medications.

The purpose of this guide is to provide you with a balanced and practical understanding of Cialis. Throughout, we'll cover everything from dosage considerations to potential side effects, best practices, and lifestyle factors that may influence its effectiveness. This guide is designed as an educational resource to support informed decision-making and effective communication with healthcare providers. However, it's essential to seek personalized advice from a medical professional to determine if Cialis is the right choice for you, based on your individual health needs.

Understanding Erectile Dysfunction (ED)

In this chapter, we explore the complexities of erectile dysfunction (ED), a condition that impacts millions of men globally. ED refers to the consistent inability to achieve or maintain an erection sufficient for satisfactory sexual activity. Though often thought of as simply a physical issue, ED can be influenced by both physiological and psychological factors and can have a profound impact on quality of life.

What Is Erectile Dysfunction?

ED is characterized by persistent difficulty with erections, but it's important to understand that it can occur for various reasons. ED may manifest occasionally or be an ongoing challenge, depending on the individual's circumstances. Notably, it is not an uncommon experience, and many men face episodes of ED at different life stages, making it a condition worth addressing with compassion and openness.

Common Causes and Factors

The causes of ED are varied, often involving a mix of physical, psychological, and lifestyle-related elements. Common physical factors include cardiovascular issues, diabetes, obesity, hormonal imbalances, and side effects from certain medications. Lifestyle factors such as smoking, alcohol consumption, lack of exercise, and poor diet can also increase the risk of ED. Additionally, stress, anxiety, depression, and relationship issues are psychological factors that frequently play a role. Understanding these causes can help men approach ED with greater awareness and identify areas for improvement or support.

What is Cialis?

In this chapter, we will discuss Cialis (tadalafil), a commonly prescribed medication for managing erectile dysfunction (ED) and benign prostatic hyperplasia (BPH) in men. Containing the active ingredient tadalafil, Cialis belongs to a category of drugs known as phosphodiesterase type 5 (PDE5) inhibitors. This medication may help increase blood flow to certain areas, making it easier to achieve and maintain an erection when there is sexual arousal.

Cialis may have a longer-lasting effect, which can last up to 36 hours. This characteristic provides more flexibility than some other medications in the same class. Additionally, Cialis has approval for treating symptoms of BPH, such as urinary challenges, offering a broader utility for those dealing with both conditions.

It is important to note that while Cialis can support physical response, it does not influence sexual desire. This medication works best when taken responsibly and with a healthcare provider's guidance, ensuring that it aligns safely with individual health considerations.

How Cialis Works In The Body

In this chapter, we will explore how Cialis works to address erectile dysfunction (ED) and benign prostatic hyperplasia (BPH). Cialis contains tadalafil, which belongs to a class of medications known as phosphodiesterase type 5 (PDE5) inhibitors.

When you take Cialis, it increases the levels of a chemical called cyclic guanosine monophosphate (cGMP) in the body. This chemical plays a crucial role in relaxing the muscles in the blood vessels of the penis, allowing for increased blood flow. This is essential for achieving and maintaining an erection during sexual arousal.

For men with BPH, Cialis helps relax the smooth muscles in the prostate and bladder, which can help ease urinary symptoms such as frequent urination, urgency, or difficulty starting a stream.

While Cialis does not directly cause arousal, it makes it easier for the body to respond to sexual stimulation. The medication's effects can last up to 36 hours, which is why it is sometimes referred to as the "weekend pill." However, it's important to remember that it only works when you are sexually stimulated, and it should be taken according to your healthcare provider's instructions to ensure safe and effective use.

Uses Of Cialis

In this chapter, we will be discussing the uses of Cialis (tadalafil)

Cialis may be prescribed for two primary conditions: erectile dysfunction (ED) and benign prostatic hyperplasia (BPH).

1. **Erectile Dysfunction (ED)**: Cialis may help men with ED achieve and maintain an erection during sexual activity by improving blood flow to the penis. It can be an option for men who have difficulty achieving or sustaining an erection.

2. **Benign Prostatic Hyperplasia (BPH)**: Cialis is also used to treat symptoms of BPH, an enlarged

prostate that can cause urinary issues such as frequent urination or difficulty starting and stopping urination. It works by relaxing muscles in the prostate and bladder.

It is important to consult with a healthcare provider before using Cialis to ensure it is an appropriate option based on individual health considerations.

Available Dosages And Forms

In this chapter, we will explore the different dosages and forms of Cialis (tadalafil), which is used to manage erectile dysfunction (ED) and benign prostatic hyperplasia (BPH).

Cialis is available in several strengths, generally in tablet form. The available doses are:

1. **2.5 mg**: This low-dose option is typically prescribed for daily use. It may be suitable for men who prefer a consistent effect for ED or BPH management without having to time the medication around sexual activity.

2. **5 mg**: A 5 mg tablet is also taken daily to address symptoms of ED or BPH. It's often used by men who experience both conditions.

3. **10 mg**: This is a common starting dose for men using Cialis on an as-needed basis. It is usually taken about 30 minutes before sexual activity. Your healthcare provider may adjust the dose based on your response.

4. **20 mg**: This higher dose may be prescribed for men who require a stronger effect or have not found relief with the 10 mg dose. It is also taken before sexual activity, typically about 30 minutes prior.

Cialis is taken orally in tablet form. It is important to follow your healthcare provider's instructions regarding the appropriate dose and timing. Your doctor may adjust the dosage depending on your individual needs and response to the medication.

How To Take Cialis

Taking Cialis correctly can help maximize its potential benefits. Here are some general guidelines:

1. **Timing and Dosage**: Cialis is available in both daily and as-needed forms. For as-needed use, it's typically taken 30 minutes before the anticipated activity, while the daily form is taken once a day at the same time. Dosage may vary based on the purpose (ED or BPH) and individual needs, so always follow the prescribed dosage.

2. **With or Without Food**: Cialis can be taken with or without food. However, heavy or high-fat meals may slightly delay the effect for some individuals.

3. **Avoiding Alcohol**: Excessive alcohol consumption can potentially lower blood pressure and may increase the risk of side effects when combined with Cialis. Limiting alcohol can help ensure the best results.

4. **Consistency**: If taking a daily dose, try to take it at the same time each day. For as-needed use, take it only when you anticipate activity.

5. **Consultation**: It's best to discuss any concerns with a healthcare provider to confirm the best dosage and frequency for individual needs. Always follow your provider's instructions on usage.

By following these practices, individuals can take steps toward a more effective experience with Cialis.

Precautions Before Using Cialis

Before using Cialis (tadalafil), there are several important factors to consider. These precautions help ensure its safe and effective use:

1. **Medical Conditions**: Certain health conditions may affect how Cialis interacts in the body. Individuals with heart problems, low blood pressure, liver or kidney issues, or any conditions affecting blood flow should consult a healthcare provider before use. Additionally, Cialis may not be suitable for those with certain eye disorders.

2. **Medication Interactions**: Some medications can interact with Cialis, potentially leading to unwanted effects. Nitrates (commonly prescribed for chest pain), alpha-blockers (for blood pressure), and certain antifungal or antibiotic medications can interact with Cialis, so it's best

to discuss any medications you're currently taking with your provider.

3. **Allergies**: If you have a known allergy to tadalafil (the active ingredient in Cialis) or any of the inactive components in the medication, it's important to avoid using it.

4. **Alcohol and Recreational Drugs**: Excessive alcohol and certain recreational drugs can increase the likelihood of side effects with Cialis. Limiting alcohol intake and avoiding recreational drugs can help reduce these risks.

5. **Age Considerations**: Cialis is primarily intended for adult use, and those over 65 may experience enhanced sensitivity. It's always recommended to discuss any age-related considerations with a healthcare provider to determine appropriate dosing.

6. **Other Lifestyle Factors**: Factors such as smoking and diet can also play a role in Cialis's effectiveness and should be considered when discussing treatment options.

By taking these precautions into account, individuals can help support a safer experience with Cialis, and open dialogue with a healthcare provider can ensure a well-informed approach.

Dietary Consideration

In this chapter, we will be discussing diets that can support the efficiency of cialis. These include:

1. **Leafy Greens**: High in nitrates to boost blood flow.

2. **Nuts & Seeds**: Provide zinc and healthy fats for hormone health.

3. **Fatty Fish**: Omega-3s support heart health.

4. **Citrus Fruits**: Vitamin C aids circulation.

5. **Berries**: Rich in antioxidants for vascular health.

6. **Watermelon**: Contains citrulline, which may help blood flow.

7. **Dark Chocolate**: Contains antioxidants that aid circulation.

A balanced diet with these foods may support overall wellness, contributing to optimal results with Cialis.

Foods And Drinks To Avoid With Cialis

In this chapter, we will be discussing foods and drinks that may interfere with how Cialis (tadalafil) is processed in the body

1. **Grapefruit**: This may interfere with how Cialis is processed in the body.

2. **High-Fat Meals**: Can delay Cialis's absorption and effectiveness.

3. **Alcohol**: Excessive drinking may reduce effectiveness and increase side effects like dizziness.

4. **Salty Foods**: High sodium intake can affect blood pressure, which is essential for Cialis to work effectively.

5. **Sugary Foods and Drinks**: Excess sugar can impact vascular health, which may influence Cialis's results.

6. **Processed Foods**: Often high in trans fats, which may impact circulation.

Limiting these foods and drinks can help support better results with Cialis while minimizing potential interactions.

Lifestyle Recommendations While Using Cialis

In this chapter, we will be discussing lifestyles that may help support the benefits of Cialis and enhance overall well-being.

1. **Exercise Regularly**: Engaging in moderate exercise, like walking, swimming, or light weightlifting, supports cardiovascular health and blood circulation, which are important for Cialis's effectiveness.

2. **Maintain a Balanced Diet**: Eating a variety of fruits, vegetables, lean proteins, and whole grains helps promote overall wellness and may enhance the body's response to Cialis.

3. **Limit Alcohol**: While occasional alcohol is usually fine, excessive drinking can lower

effectiveness and increase side effects like dizziness or low blood pressure.

4. **Manage Stress**: Chronic stress can interfere with sexual performance. Practices like deep breathing, meditation, and mindfulness can help reduce stress levels.

5. **Get Enough Sleep**: Aiming for 7–8 hours of quality sleep each night supports hormonal balance and energy, both of which are crucial for optimal Cialis results.

6. **Avoid Smoking**: Smoking can negatively impact blood flow, so reducing or quitting smoking may improve Cialis's effectiveness.

Common Side Effects Of Cialis

In this chapter, we will discuss the common side effects of Cialis. It is important to discuss with your doctor if you notice any side effects after using Cialis.

1. **Headaches**: some users may experience headaches often mild to moderate.

2. **Indigestion and Heartburn**: Some users may experience digestive discomfort.

3. **Back Pain and Muscle Aches**: Typically mild, sometimes occurring a day or two after use.

4. **Nasal Congestion**: Some users experience a stuffy nose.

5. **Flushing**: Warmth or redness, often noticeable on the face and neck.

6. **Dizziness**: Mild dizziness may be reported by some users.

These side effects are generally manageable, and experiences may vary based on individual responses to the medication. Discuss with your doctor, if symptoms persist.

Serious Side Effects And Allergic Reactions To Cialis

These reactions, though rare, can be serious and may require prompt medical evaluation.

1. **Chest Pain or Pressure**: This could indicate a serious issue and warrants immediate medical attention.

2. **Vision Changes or Sudden Vision Loss**: Rare but severe, this side effect can impact one or both eyes and may signal a condition known as non-arteritic anterior ischemic optic neuropathy (NAION).

3. **Hearing Loss or Ringing in the Ears**: A sudden decrease or loss of hearing is possible in some cases and may require prompt consultation.

4. **Severe Dizziness or Fainting**: This can be a sign of low blood pressure and may require medical assistance, especially if persistent.

5. **Prolonged or Painful Erection (Priapism)**: An erection lasting more than 4 hours is considered a medical emergency to prevent long-term damage.

6. **Allergic Reactions**: Some may experience hives, swelling of the face, lips, or throat, or difficulty breathing. Any signs of an allergic reaction require immediate medical attention.

Managing Side Effects Of Cialis

Always follow your healthcare provider's guidance for managing side effects, and contact them if you experience any persistent or severe reactions.

1. **Headaches**: Stay hydrated and rest in a quiet, dark room. Consult with a healthcare provider.

2. **Flushing**: Avoid alcohol and hot drinks, which can worsen flushing.

3. **Nasal Congestion**: Use a saline nasal spray or over-the-counter decongestants. Avoid using nasal sprays for long periods to prevent rebound congestion.

4. **Prolonged Erection (Priapism)**: If an erection lasts more than 4 hours, seek emergency medical help immediately.

5. **Vision Changes**: If you notice any vision changes, contact your healthcare provider immediately.

6. **Hearing Loss**: If you experience sudden hearing loss or ringing in the ears, discontinue use and consult a healthcare provider immediately.

7. **Allergic Reactions**: If you experience swelling of the face, lips, or throat, or difficulty breathing, seek emergency medical attention immediately.

Cialis Drug Interactions

Cialis may interact with certain medications and substances, potentially affecting its efficacy or increasing the risk of side effects. Here are some important interactions to consider:

1. **Nitrates**: Combining Cialis with nitrates (e.g., nitroglycerin) used for chest pain can cause a drop in blood pressure. Always inform your healthcare provider if you're using nitrates.

2. **Alpha-blockers**: Medications like doxazosin or tamsulosin, used for high blood pressure or BPH, can cause low blood pressure when combined with Cialis. Your healthcare provider may adjust your dosage or recommend an alternative.

3. **Other Erectile Dysfunction Medications**: Do not take Cialis with other ED medications (like sildenafil or vardenafil) as it can lead to an increased risk of side effects.

4. **Antibiotics and Antifungals**: Certain antibiotics (like clarithromycin) and antifungals (such as ketoconazole) can increase the level of Cialis in your bloodstream, potentially enhancing its effects or side effects.

5. **HIV Protease Inhibitors**: Drugs used to treat HIV (e.g., ritonavir, indinavir) may also increase Cialis levels, which may lead to an increased risk of side effects.

6. **Blood Pressure Medications**: Some blood pressure medications can interact with Cialis, either increasing or decreasing its effectiveness. Always inform your doctor about any blood pressure medications you are taking.

7. **Alcohol**: Excessive alcohol consumption can increase the risk of side effects like dizziness or low blood pressure when taking Cialis. Moderate alcohol intake is recommended.

8. **Grapefruit**: Grapefruit and grapefruit juice may interfere with the metabolism of Cialis, leading to an increased level of the drug in your bloodstream. It's advisable to avoid grapefruit while taking Cialis.

9. **Antacids**: Some antacids (e.g., aluminum hydroxide, magnesium hydroxide) may reduce the absorption of Cialis, potentially making it less effective.

10. **Herbal Supplements**: Supplements such as St. John's Wort, ginseng, or other herbs may affect how Cialis works or interact with other medications you're taking. Always check with a healthcare provider before adding new supplements to your routine.

Consulting Your Healthcare Provider on Potential Risks

Before starting Cialis or combining it with other medications, over-the-counter drugs, or supplements, it is crucial to consult with your healthcare provider. They can assess your medical history and current medications, ensuring that any potential drug interactions are avoided, and help you determine the safest approach for your treatment. Always inform your healthcare provider of all the medications you are taking, including OTC products and supplements, to avoid complications.

Before starting Cialis, always inform your healthcare provider about all medications, supplements, and any health conditions you have to avoid potential interactions.

Health Tests To Consider Before Starting Cialis

Before beginning Cialis, it's important to undergo certain health tests to ensure it's safe and appropriate for your individual health needs. These tests help your healthcare provider assess your overall health and manage any potential risks. Here are key tests to consider:

1. **Blood Pressure Check**: Cialis can affect blood pressure, and if you have low blood pressure or take medications that lower it, a blood pressure test is essential. This ensures that taking Cialis won't cause any harmful drops in your blood pressure.

2. **Cardiovascular Health Assessment**: Since Cialis works by improving blood flow, a cardiovascular evaluation may be necessary, especially for individuals with heart disease or a

history of cardiovascular issues. Your doctor may recommend an electrocardiogram (ECG) or other heart health tests to assess your heart function.

3. **Kidney and Liver Function Tests**: Cialis is processed by the liver and kidneys, so if you have preexisting liver or kidney conditions, these tests can help ensure that your organs can handle the medication. Your healthcare provider may adjust the dosage based on the results.

4. **Sexual Health Evaluation**: If you are experiencing erectile dysfunction, a sexual health evaluation can help identify the underlying cause, whether it's psychological, hormonal, or physical. This may involve blood tests to check for hormone levels, such as testosterone.

5. **Blood Sugar Levels**: If you have diabetes or are at risk of it, your healthcare may check your blood sugar levels. Diabetes can contribute to erectile dysfunction, and Cialis may interact with medications used to manage diabetes.

6. **Eye Health Examination**: Though rare, Cialis has been associated with changes in vision. If you have a history of eye problems or conditions like retinitis pigmentosa, an eye health check may be recommended before starting Cialis.

7. **Prostate Health Check**: For men with symptoms of benign prostatic hyperplasia (BPH) or those who are older, a prostate health test can help evaluate the severity of prostate issues. Cialis may also be used for BPH, and understanding the prostate's condition is important for effective treatment.

These tests provide a comprehensive overview of your health, ensuring that Cialis is a safe and effective treatment option. Always consult with your healthcare provider before starting Cialis, as they can advise you on the necessary tests and help monitor your health while using the medication.

Age-Specific Considerations For Cialis Use

When it comes to using Cialis for erectile dysfunction (ED) or benign prostatic hyperplasia (BPH), age can influence how effective and safe the medication is. Here's a look at some important points related to age and Cialis use:

1. Cialis for Younger Adults (Under 40)

Cialis is not typically the first choice for younger men experiencing ED, as the cause may often be related to psychological factors, stress, or lifestyle. It's important to understand the root cause of ED before considering Cialis as a treatment.

Younger individuals should consult a healthcare provider to explore the underlying factors contributing to ED and determine whether Cialis is suitable.

2. Cialis for Middle-Aged Adults (40–60)

Cialis may be a useful option for men in this age group who experience age-related ED. In some cases, lifestyle factors such as stress or physical health issues can contribute to ED, and Cialis can help improve symptoms.

Before using Cialis, it's important to consider any existing health conditions that could affect the treatment's safety or effectiveness. Regular check-ins with a healthcare provider can help monitor any changes.

3. Cialis for Older Adults (Over 60)

As men age, conditions like reduced blood flow or hormonal changes can contribute to ED. Cialis may help improve erectile function, but older adults may need dosage adjustments based on individual health conditions.

It's important to monitor health regularly, particularly for conditions like heart disease or diabetes, which can affect Cialis use. Adjusting the dose may be necessary depending on individual health status.

General Tips for All Age Groups

- **Consulting a Healthcare Provider**: Regardless of age, it's always important to consult a healthcare provider before starting Cialis. They can offer advice on how it fits into your overall health and any potential interactions with other medications.

- **Side Effects**: Age can affect how the body reacts to medications like Cialis. Some people may experience side effects differently, so staying informed and following guidelines is important for safe use.

In summary, while Cialis can be effective for many individuals, age and health status are key factors in determining how it works. It's important to consult with a healthcare provider to ensure it's the right choice for your needs.

Best Practices For Effective And Safe Cialis Use

When using Cialis, it's essential to follow best practices to ensure it is both effective and safe. This medication can help improve erectile function or manage symptoms of benign prostatic hyperplasia (BPH) when used correctly. Here are key guidelines to maximize its benefits while minimizing risks:

1. Consult a Healthcare Provider

- **Personalized Advice**: Before starting Cialis, speak with a healthcare provider. They can assess your overall health, medical history, and specific needs. A tailored plan ensures you're using the right dosage and form of Cialis.

- **Regular Check-ups**: Regular consultations with your healthcare provider help monitor your response to the medication and identify any side effects or interactions early.

2. Follow the Recommended Dosage

- **Start with the Prescribed Dose**: Stick to the dosage recommended by your doctor. Dosage typically ranges from 2.5 mg to 20 mg, depending on the individual's condition and response to the medication.

- **Avoid Overuse**: Don't exceed the recommended dose, as this may increase the risk of side effects. Taking more than prescribed will not necessarily improve effectiveness and could lead to complications.

3. Take Cialis as Directed

- **Timing and Frequency**: Cialis can be taken daily or on an as-needed basis. For daily use, a low-dose version (2.5 mg to 5 mg) is typically prescribed. For occasional use, take it 30 minutes to 1 hour before sexual activity.

- **Avoid Alcohol**: Drinking excessive amounts of alcohol can interfere with the effectiveness of Cialis and increase the risk of side effects.

Limiting alcohol intake is advisable while using the medication.

4. Avoid Certain Foods and Drinks

- **High-Fat Meals**: Consuming heavy, fatty meals before taking Cialis can delay the absorption of the medication. Try to avoid large, high-fat meals around the time you plan to take Cialis.

- **Limit Grapefruit**: Grapefruit can interact with certain medications, including Cialis, affecting their efficacy. It is best to limit or avoid grapefruit and its juice.

5. Monitor for Side Effects

- **Stay Alert to Any Changes**: While Cialis is generally well-tolerated, be aware of potential side effects such as headaches, indigestion, or dizziness. If you experience unusual symptoms or persistent side effects, contact your healthcare provider.

- **Serious Reactions**: Although rare, serious side effects like chest pain, vision changes, or an erection lasting longer than 4 hours (priapism) require immediate medical attention.

6. Use Cialis with Caution if You Have Certain Conditions

- **Pre-existing Health Issues**: If you have heart disease, low blood pressure, or other chronic conditions, inform your healthcare provider before using Cialis. These conditions may require dose adjustments or alternative treatments.

- **Medication Interactions**: Avoid taking Cialis with certain medications, particularly nitrates (often used for chest pain) or medications for high blood pressure, as these can cause dangerous drops in blood pressure.

7. Lifestyle Adjustments for Better Results

- **Healthy Habits**: A balanced diet, regular exercise, and maintaining a healthy weight can improve the effectiveness of Cialis. Additionally, managing stress, avoiding smoking, and limiting alcohol intake can have a positive impact on erectile function.

- **Mental Health Matters**: Psychological factors such as stress or anxiety can affect erectile function. Seeking support from a therapist or counselor, if needed, may improve outcomes alongside Cialis use.

Always remember, that personalized guidance from a healthcare provider is key to using Cialis appropriately.

Understanding Cialis Tolerance and Resistance

In this chapter, we will be discussing Cialis tolerance and resistance.

Tolerance to Cialis

Tolerance refers to the process where the body gradually becomes less responsive to medication over time, requiring higher doses to achieve the same effect.

- **Rare with Cialis**: Unlike certain medications, tolerance to Cialis is not commonly observed. Most individuals will continue to experience the same level of effectiveness with the prescribed dosage over the long term.

- **Factors that May Influence Tolerance**: factors such as age, overall health, and other medications may impact how well the drug works. For example, someone with underlying health conditions like heart disease or diabetes may find that their response to Cialis changes over time.

- **Adjusting Dosage**: If an individual feels that Cialis is becoming less effective, it's essential to consult with a healthcare provider. Adjusting the dosage or exploring alternative treatments may help.

Resistance to Cialis

Resistance typically refers to the body's diminished response to a medication, often due to adaptive changes in the body or underlying conditions. In the case of Cialis, resistance is generally not a concern, as it works by increasing blood flow to the penis through the inhibition of the enzyme phosphodiesterase type 5 (PDE5).

- Resistance to Cialis is rare because its action mechanism doesn't usually lead to the body adapting in a way that reduces its effectiveness.

- **Potential Contributing Factors**: While Cialis resistance is unlikely, factors such as poor cardiovascular health, certain medications, or other medical conditions may reduce the effectiveness of Cialis. These factors may make it appear as if resistance is developing when in fact, the underlying cause lies elsewhere.

When to Seek Professional Guidance

If you feel that Cialis is no longer as effective as it once was, it's crucial to consult a healthcare provider to rule out underlying health conditions or adjust your treatment plan. They can assess:

- **Underlying Health Conditions**: Conditions such as diabetes, high blood pressure, or cardiovascular disease may affect the effectiveness of Cialis.

- **Medication Interactions**: Some medications may interfere with Cialis, making it less effective.

- **Psychological Factors**: Mental health issues like stress or anxiety can impact erectile function and reduce the perceived effectiveness of Cialis.

It is essential to stay aware of the potential impact of tolerance and other factors on its effectiveness. Regular communication with a healthcare provider ensures that the medication remains effective and suitable for your specific needs.

Proper Storage And Handling of Cialis

Storing Cialis (tadalafil) properly is essential to ensure its effectiveness and safety. Mismanagement of the medication can lead to reduced potency or contamination, impacting its intended use. To maintain the medication's quality, proper storage and handling should be prioritized.

Cialis should be stored at room temperature, typically between 68°F and 77°F (20°C and 25°C). It is essential to keep the medication in a cool, dry environment. Exposure to high humidity or extreme temperatures can degrade the medication. It should also be kept away from direct light, which can further compromise its integrity. For the best results, Cialis should be stored in its original container, sealed tightly to protect it from moisture and light.

Another critical aspect is ensuring that Cialis is kept out of reach of children and pets. It is advisable to store the medication in a secure place, such as a locked cabinet or high shelf, to prevent accidental ingestion. Additionally, it is important to check the expiration date on the packaging regularly. Using expired medication can be ineffective and possibly unsafe. Any unused or expired Cialis should be disposed of properly, following local disposal guidelines, to avoid environmental harm or accidental ingestion.

Handling Cialis requires adherence to the prescribed instructions. The tablets should not be crushed, split, or chewed, as this could alter their effectiveness. Only take the prescribed dose, and never combine Cialis with other erectile dysfunction medications without consulting a healthcare provider, as doing so can cause harmful interactions.

In conclusion, proper storage and handling of Cialis are essential for maintaining its efficacy and safety. By storing the medication correctly, checking expiration dates, and following usage guidelines, individuals can ensure they are using Cialis effectively for its intended purpose. If in doubt, consult a healthcare professional or pharmacist for further advice on safe storage and disposal practices.

Health Monitoring While Using Cialis

1. **Blood Pressure Monitoring**

   Regularly check your blood pressure to ensure it remains within a safe range. Cialis may lower blood pressure, especially when combined with other medications like nitrates.

2. **Side Effect Awareness**

   Monitor for common side effects like headaches, dizziness, or digestive issues. If symptoms persist or worsen, consult your healthcare provider for advice.

3. **Pre-existing Health Conditions**

   Individuals with heart, liver, or kidney issues should be closely monitored. These conditions may affect how your body processes Cialis, requiring dose adjustments or extra care.

4. **Effectiveness Tracking**

Keep track of how well Cialis is working for you. If you're not experiencing the expected results, discuss potential changes to your treatment plan with your healthcare provider.

5. **Kidney and Liver Function**

For those with kidney or liver problems, regular tests may be needed to monitor how Cialis is being metabolized and ensure safe use.

6. **Adjustments for Older Adults**

Older individuals may need closer monitoring due to slower metabolism. Regular consultations with a healthcare provider are crucial for safe use.

7. **Monitoring Drug Interactions**

Be aware of any new medications, supplements, or changes in your treatment. Certain drugs may interact with Cialis and affect its efficacy or cause side effects.

By regularly monitoring these factors and maintaining communication with your healthcare provider, you can safely use Cialis and ensure its effectiveness in managing erectile dysfunction.

Creating A Sustainable Approach To Sexual Health

A sustainable approach to sexual health considers more than just immediate solutions—it's about building habits and making choices that support long-term well-being. This involves maintaining a balanced lifestyle that prioritizes physical health, mental wellness, and open communication.

Physical health is fundamental. Regular exercise, a nutritious diet, and sufficient sleep all contribute to a body that's well-prepared for intimacy. Exercise, particularly, enhances circulation, which is essential for sexual function, while a balanced diet can provide the nutrients needed to support energy and hormone balance. Avoiding excessive alcohol, smoking, and recreational drug use also plays a significant role, as these can negatively impact sexual health.

Mental wellness is equally crucial. Managing stress, anxiety, and depression through therapy, meditation, or other coping strategies can help address issues that often underlie sexual health concerns. It's important to keep in mind that sexual health is not just physical; emotional health, self-esteem, and a positive body image all contribute to an individual's comfort and satisfaction in their intimate life.

Communication with partners is another key aspect of a sustainable sexual health approach. Open, honest conversations about needs, boundaries, and expectations can enhance connection and mutual understanding. This emotional closeness often reinforces trust and reduces performance anxiety.

Ultimately, a sustainable approach means taking steps that support sexual health in a balanced, ongoing way, creating a foundation that benefits not only intimacy but overall quality of life.

Conclusion

Erectile dysfunction (ED) is a common but often complex challenge that can impact various aspects of life, from self-confidence to relationships. This guide has offered insights into managing ED with the help of Cialis, aiming to provide you with clear, practical information to make informed decisions.

We've explored how Cialis works, discussed its different dosage options, explained potential side effects, and highlighted the importance of understanding interactions with other medications. We also touched on lifestyle considerations and realistic expectations, emphasizing a balanced approach.

It's important to have open communication with a healthcare provider, considering all factors from dosage to potential interactions. Remember that this guide is a resource, and while it covers the fundamentals, your healthcare provider can offer personalized advice tailored to your unique situation.

Made in the USA
Monee, IL
18 November 2024

70419448R00036